7 Foolproof Steps to Lose the Baby Weight in 6 Months or Less

VIRGINIA MARTIN

DEDICATION

Dedicated to all the mothers.

CONTENTS

INTRODUCTION

Hello, beautiful Mama! I'm so glad you've picked up this copy of *7 Foolproof Steps to Lose the Baby Weight in 6 Months or Less!* You're about to begin a journey that will leave you feeling stronger, more energetic, happier and more grounded. Seriously.

I know that's a lot to promise but I can tell you from personal experience: these seven steps work. I know because this is exactly the process I followed to lose the 40 lbs within 6 months of giving birth.

Let me tell you: losing weight doesn't have to be the terrible, deprivation-laden process we've all gotten to know so well through countless weight loss books and schemes. Instead, it can be a nourishing, rejuvenating process that leaves you feeling ten times more vibrant than when you started.

Isn't that refreshing?

So here's the deal: weight loss can be a tricky – and deeply personal – topic. I encourage you to be gentle with yourself; be exceptionally kind, because you've only got one you... and your baby only has one Mama! Not to mention that there *is* a secret ingredient that speeds weight loss along big time: your attitude.

Yep. Your mental approach to this whole thing will seriously impact the results you see.

When you embrace the process and *love yourself through it*, you'll see faster results. I can't stress this enough: your body *is you*. The things you think *affect your body directly.*

Don't worry – we'll get more into this a bit later. But for now, let's dig in to the easiest, most safe and loving way to lose weight – ever.

To your healthy + vibrant life,

Virginia

1 HOW TO USE THIS BOOK

Change takes time. It took 9 months to gain the weight, and it's not going to all come off at once!

Have patience – this process works if you let it.

But I'll let you in on a little secret: while all these steps are important to reshaping your body, the real key is to feel good and find your joy.

Yes! That's right – when women are happy, they're much more likely to feel good about themselves, open themselves to fun, new experiences, and release weight and food dependencies.

Every step I outline in this book is going to bring you closer to the fun, loving life that you crave – and losing the weight is just part of the bigger picture.

You don't need to implement all these steps at once. In fact, I encourage you to take a few at a time and integrate them into your life. Some will be easy for you, others will be more difficult; everyone is different.

But believe me: there is a wonderful, joy-filled life waiting for you to step up to the plate and embrace it.

2 THE DON'TS

Let's start with a few very, very important ground rules in our process. There are some things that you might be tempted to try during your weight loss journey that I can tell you straight up won't work.

And worse... they could sabotage your efforts big time.

There are only a handful of don'ts, beautiful Mama. If you can keep them at bay you'll be ten steps ahead of the game.

Don't Diet

You might be tempted to pair these steps with some kind of funky, trendy diet like South Beach, Atkins, Paleo, or some other wack-a-doodle "in-style" diet. Don't do it!

Do I really have to remind you that diets don't work? They don't. They really, really, don't. If they did, there wouldn't be so many endless books about weight loss out there because everyone would have just figured it out when they tried the diet in the first place.

Diets don't work because...

> ...they cause you to feel deprived, which leads to overeating and binge eating.

...they most often keep you on a restricted rotation of food, which is boring and you'll eventually lose interest.

...they are dependent on "will power," which is a great thing in the short run, but in the long run, "will power" burns out and you'll go back to doing what you're doing now.

Don't Kill Yourself with Exercise

You may also be tempted to jump headlong into a radical exercise class or exercise schedule – please don't do that! Biting off more than your body is ready to handle is the most common way people become injured (trust me, I've been there, and I've seen many, many other people go through this process).

We'll talk more about exercise in the 7 Steps, but please take a deep breath and realize that you really don't need to kill yourself with exercise to lose weight. It's not about punishing your body, so leave the marathon treadmill sessions and back-breaking (literally) Cross-Fit sessions for another day.

Trust me: this process works. And it *does not* involve horrendous, make-you-wanna-puke exercise-til-you-die.

Don't Drink Soda

Okay, okay – this is the one change that may be difficult for you soda drinkers. Any kind of sugary food that you consume on a daily basis is going to be a major contributor to weight gain (or lack of weight loss). Soda is the number one culprit – and also the easiest thing to cut from your diet.

If you're a regular soda drinker, even if it's "diet" (and by the way, "diet" soda is so much worse for you than regular), let's work on curbing that bad habit.

Here are some things you can do to cut down your soda intake:

- Notice how many sodas you drink on a daily basis. Let's see if we can half that number. So if you normally have 4 Cokes in a day, can you cut it down to 2? Give it a shot!

- Switch to regular. Seriously. I know you'll probably think I'm crazy, but there's science behind this: fake sugars are linked to heart disease, stroke, diabetes, obesity, high cholesterol, osteoporosis, liver damage and kidney stones. Not to mention... it's terrible for Baby if you're breast-feeding.

- If you're drinking a dark soda, like Coke, transition to a light-colored soda if you can.

- Best case scenario, you'll drink fizzy water instead – perhaps even cut the sparkling water with fruit juice like cranberry, orange or grapefruit! This way you'll still get a sweet, fizzy drink without the tablespoons of sugar or nasty fake sweeteners.

That's it for the don'ts – there are only three, and if you can manage to do all of them, you're way ahead of the game, Mama!

3 STEP 1: WATER
DRINK HALF YOUR BODY WEIGHT IN WATER EACH DAY

Water makes all the difference.

Water helps the body flush toxins, it helps you eliminate and reduce bloating, it helps your skin look plump and lustrous, and it is incredibly energizing. We were made to depend on water, so give your body what it wants!

Dehydration can cause so many frustrating symptoms: headache, bloat, constipation, dry/wrinkled skin, acne, lack of energy... and so many more.

Isn't it amazing that all these things can be cured just by getting enough water in your system?

How Much Water to Drink

As a guideline, plan to drink half your body weight in ounces of water every day.

So, if you weight 150 lbs, plan to drink 75 oz. of water every day.

At first, this may feel like a lot (and yeah, you might be peeing quite frequently! Don't worry, your body will adjust), but you will soon find that common ailments that were troubling you have disappeared.

I use a glass jug or water bottle that has ounces marked on it. Every morning I fill it up and throughout the day I either pour the water into a cup if I'm at work or drink directly from the jug if I'm out and about. This way, I can easily measure how much water I've had that day and make sure I'm keeping up.

Quality of Water Matters

If possible, it's best to drink filtered water. If you can't get a filter installed directly on your tap, I suggest picking up a Brita Filter to make sure your water is as clean as possible.

A quick note: we've been hearing a lot about problems with single-use plastic bottles. Not only are they wrecking havoc on our environment, but chemicals in the plastic actually leach into the water and are then absorbed into your body (yikes!). This can affect your weight loss process as well as the health of your baby, especially if the plastic was heated (as in a hot car).

Never drink out of a hot single-use plastic water bottle if you can help it, and avoid re-filling a single-use plastic water bottle as well.

In fact, it's best to avoid them altogether.

Try and get a glass water bottle or jug or at least make sure that your reusable plastic water bottle is BPA-free. BPA-free plastic is relatively easy to find these days... but glass is still best.

Replace Soda with Water

If you're one of my soda-drinking gals, consider replacing at least one of your daily sodas with clear, refreshing water. You'll feel a difference pretty quickly – once you get over your sugar withdrawal, that is!

Action Steps

We are so lucky to have access to clean drinking water. Take advantage of this and drink up, Mama! Here are steps you can take today to get started:

1. Figure out how much water you need to drink on the daily. Your body weight ÷ 2 = the number of ounces of water you should have every day.
2. Get a glass jug or BPA-free reusable plastic water bottle and use it every day to measure your water intake.

Quick Tip: When you wake up in the morning, have 8 ounces of water to get your day started. Avoid drinking too much water before going to bed... you'll be up to use the restroom before too long!

4 STEP 2: THE OUTDOORS
GO OUTSIDE AT LEAST ONCE A DAY

Depending on where you live – and how you live – this might be the easiest step... or the hardest!

I recently read that modern Americans spend 90% of their time indoors. Can you believe it!? What happened to the days when children would play outdoors and the family would sit on the back deck and gaze into the fading daylight to wind down the day? Television and screens have replaced much of our outdoor time... but that doesn't mean it's not still important.

When there are children in your life, spending time outside becomes, generally, easier. Take the baby for a walk outside or simply sit on the front steps for a few minutes to watch people passing by.

Of course, during the cold winter months it becomes harder to go outside – but that just means you can bundle up and play in the snow!

Vitamin D Improves Mood

When the sun hits our skin, our mood is scientifically proven to lift. And guess what happens when your mood lifts? You're easier to be around, you're more playful, and suddenly that afternoon indoors with a bucket of ice cream doesn't seem like the "reward" you were thinking it would be.

Being Outdoors Gets the Body Moving

Outdoor activities tend to involve more movement: gardening, walking, pushing a stroller, etc. More movement improves mood, burns more calories, and keeps your body flexible and strong.

Fresh Air is Invigorating

Ever spent the entire day inside and felt completely energized and renewed when you walked outdoors? This is why a brisk walk around the block can clear your head, help you get fresh ideas and re-center and ground you so well.

Okay, Mama, I think I know what's going through your head right now... you're wondering, "How in the hell is spending 20 minutes outdoors each day going to help me lose weight!?"

Well, it will – indirectly. It will help lift you mood, give you more energy, and reconnect with the wide world. Those are all important things if you want to lose weight.

When a woman gets to her healthiest weight – and is able to maintain it – it's not because she sat inside all day. It's not because she counted calories and weighed out every single portion of food she consumed. It's not because she agonized over the number on the scale. It's not because she killed herself every day with mind-numbing exercise. It's not because she dieted.

It's because she *lived her life*. She laughed, she did things she loves, she felt good in her body... and she went outside to enjoy the beautiful world!

Action Items

1. Think of three things you could do outside. Maybe it's drawing with sidewalk chalk with a child, maybe it's walking to the post office, maybe it's going for a bike ride. Find three excuses to get outside the house!
2. Commit to going outside for at least 20 minutes today... and then, do it!

Quick Tip: Don't forget sunscreen for you and Baby!

5 STEP 3: SLEEP
GET AT LEAST 8 HOURS OF SLEEP PER DAY

Okay – I *know* you're rolling your eyes at me over this one! When you have a new baby, it's incredibly difficult to get a full, uninterrupted night of sleep – I get it!

But here's the thing...

In study after study after study, weight loss participants who get about eight hours of sleep per night lose significantly more weight than those who get six hours of sleep per night.

Ever had the chance to sleep through the night and wake up on your own, aka, without an alarm? Did you notice how fit and slim you felt the next morning?

Your body requires sleep to process food, eliminate toxins and "reset." When you sleep more, you lose more weight.

And guess what? Those eight hours don't have to be consecutive.

Yes – that means that you can get the same benefit from sleeping in bursts throughout the day!

So, take every opportunity to snag a nap whether that's on your lunch break if you're back at work, or in the afternoon while Baby is snoozing.

Many women think it's a good idea to get chores done while the baby is asleep, which means that they never get rest time. Take a cue from Baby and get some Zzz's while the little one is out.

Take Turns with Dad

If Dad is in the picture, see if you can switch off nights – on Monday night, you wake with the baby, on Tuesday night, he wakes with the baby, and so on. If you're breast-feeding, make sure you have pumped enough to feed the baby.

Take Advantage of Sleep Tips

There are a few basic things you can do to improve your sleep.

- Avoid screens toward the end of the day. The blue light emitted from phones, computers and tablets signals to your brain that it's early morning and your body will respond by becoming more alert, making it difficult to fall asleep.
- Avoid caffeine after 3 pm. Also, if you take vitamins as a supplement, be aware that Vitamin B12 can keep you awake and should be avoided after 3 pm.
- Create a gentle, nourishing nighttime routine for yourself to wind down as the day ends, signaling your body that it's time to sleep.

Action Steps

It's pretty simple (but not necessarily easy!): make sleep a priority. The dishes can be done later, but if you don't take advantage of your opportunities to sleep, your body will hold on to weight like whoa!

6 STEP 4: GREEN MEALS
REPLACE ONE MEAL A DAY WITH A "GREEN MEAL"

It's so easy to get in the habit of eating pre-packaged foods that sometimes we give up our veggies in lieu of easy-to-grab microwavables (or worse – fast food!).

Look, I know that it's not realistic to expect that you can eat super healthy "perfect" meals three times a day. That's not real life! Real life is messy, it's sometimes frantic and often overwhelming.

So here's what I'm asking: every day replace one meal with a big, crispy, leafy green salad. I suggest replacing lunch.

Oh – and just to be clear, I'm not talking about boring iceberg lettuce salads that take forever to wash, chop and then clean the colander afterwards. No way! Who has time for that?

I'm talking about lush, nutrient-dense, vitamin-packed super food salads that you can throw together in five minutes.

Here's how it works...

Purchase Ready-to-Eat Greens

Wherever you do your grocery shopping, select pre-washed greens to seriously cut down on your salad-making time. I personally love to shop at Trader Joe's, but pretty much every grocer has ready-to-eat greens in the produce section.

Whenever I'm shopping for the week, I'll get a bucket of spinach, pre-cut kale, arugula and romaine lettuce and keep it in the fridge for easy-to-throw-together salads during the week.

Switch to Oils

Salad dressings are great but I think they can get boring. Instead, I prefer to use a simple olive oil on my salads (or sesame oil) and put all the pizazz into the toppings.

Keep Healthy Toppings Around

Almonds, cashews, pine nuts, pistachios, macadamia nuts, sunflower seeds, golden raisins, ground flaxseeds and toasted sesame seeds and just some of my favorite salad toppings. To me, the toppings keep things really exciting – and every week when I'm shopping I'll pick up a new slew of them!

If you can eat dairy, it's also fun to put cheese on top – I love parmesan, feta and Jarlsburg.

Don't forget the salt and pepper! On my kale salads I also love to add paprika – and don't be shy about experimenting with other veggies as well. Corn, chopped bell peppers and onions are always a nice touch.

Action Steps

When you shop this week, add some greens to your cart. Commit to replacing one meal a day with a beautiful salad!

SALAD RECIPES

Kale Delight

Ingredients

- Chopped Kale
- Olive Oil
- Toasted Almonds
- Parmesan Cheese
- Salt & Pepper

Place chopped kale in a bowl. Pour on as much olive oil as you like, and then massage it into the leaves. Top with almonds, cheese and salt & pepper.

Arugula Explosion

Ingredients

- Arugula
- Olive Oil
- Golden Raisins
- Macadamia Nuts
- Romano Cheese
- Salt & Pepper

Place arugula in a bowl. Top with olive oil, adding toppings.

Keepin' It Simple with Romaine

Ingredients

- Romaine Lettuce
- Balsamic Vinaigrette Dressing
- Feta Cheese
- Chopped Strawberries

Mix all ingredients in bowl.

7 STEP 5: SEX!
HAVE SEX AT LEAST ONCE A WEEK

Just because you're a Mama now doesn't mean the sex has to stop! You're not just any Mama – you're a *hot Mama* – and the sooner you believe and embrace it yourself, the more sex you'll be having and the quicker the weight will fall off.

Regular sexual activity has tremendous benefits for women and men, but here are just a few benefits you'll see...

Sex is Exercise

We're looking for any reason to get moving more, and sex is a *great* way to get your blood flowing, get your heart pounding and awaken your body!

The More You Have, the More You Want

Besides increased activity levels, when a woman has regular sex she feels sexier. And when she feels sexier in her day-to-day life, she's much less likely to go through the drive-thru and binge on the fries.

Listen, I get it: when you've got weight to lose, it's harder to feel interested in sex... and yes, libido even goes down when you're carrying extra weight.

But let's get one thing straight – your man loves your body. He's interested, trust me. If you start putting out signals, I can almost guarantee that he'll respond positively and you can get it on.

Funnily enough, despite the fact that sex is such an important part of a healthy adult's life, sex is one area in which we women tend to get hung up. We think, "Oh, once I lose the weight, *then* I'll feel sexy and I'll want to have sex."

But actually, it's the other way around! When you accept and love yourself – extra weight and all – you'll feel more free to enjoy sex, and the weight will fall off more naturally.

Action Steps

Go ahead, enjoy it! Schedule a sex session if you have to – but find a time to get in between the sheets with your hubby A.S.A.P.

You know what? If you don't have time even for a quickie, I dare you to pull your man aside and give him a nice, slow, sensual kiss the next time you see him. That ought to shake things up a bit! Try it and see what happens.

Quick Tip: Don't forget... just because you so recently had a baby doesn't mean you can't get pregnant again almost right away. One of my girlfriends thought she couldn't get pregnant right after giving birth... now she has Irish twins!

8 STEP 6: EXERCISE
EXERCISE 3-4 TIMES PER WEEK

Ah. We've finally gotten to the portion of the book where we talk about the most feared and loathed aspect of weight loss.

Exercise.

But you already know that I am NOT a fan of ass-kicking, "sweat until you puke" workouts. No way! In fact, I am decidedly *against* those kinds of workouts.

In fact, I am against anything that makes you hate exercising.

Here's what exercise should look like in your life:

3-4 times per week spend an hour or so working on your body. This might be slow, meditative yoga classes that lengthen your limbs and create centered strength. It might be a challenging barre class at a studio like The Bar Method that is known for exercises that are super safe (developed with a physical therapist) to create beautiful muscle definition. It might be an hour of swimming in the pool, getting your heart rate up without wrecking your joints.

Here's what exercise *should never, ever look like:*

- Hours of painful cardio that leaves you feeling depleted and starving.

- Running for extended periods of time on concrete, which will destroy your joints.
- Doing quick, jerky movements with heavy weights that can seriously pull muscles, throw out backs and even cause you to permanently damage joints and ligaments.
- Anything that leaves you feeling like you "hate" exercise.

Everyone is different and every body needs something a little different as well. If a brisk mile-long walk down the beach is your jam, that's perfect! If you like to do the elliptical machine and then lift some weights, great. If you play tennis with friends, perfect.

Your exercise habit should be something that you can consistently maintain... because it's fun, it's safe, and when you're done, you *feel good!*

Action Items:

- Try a new class that seems interesting. Many cities have something called "Class Pass" where you pay a flat monthly fee and you can try classes at different studios or gyms in the area. A good way to explore new things!
- Get moving 3-4 times a week to really see changes start to happen.

9 STEP 7: MINDSET
MAKE A MINDSET SHIFT

When you love your body, it will love you back. The most important thing you can do to change your body is to love it through the changes – and that may mean it's time for a big mindset shift!

Think about it: do you catch yourself thinking things like, "I wish I weren't so fat," or "I hate my thighs," or "I look like a whale"?

Those thoughts affect your body. Remember what I said earlier – you *are* your body. Your body is a direct outward reflection of what is going on inside your mind. So every time you eat something and feel guilty about it, or feel shame for not exercising, or start saying terrible things to yourself in your head, you're only reinforcing the extra weight and an unhappy situation.

So the big question becomes... how can you shift your mindset into a more positive, life-affirming one?

Gratitude

Believe me... I've been in the downward spiral. I've been in that place where you feel so awful about yourself that things get worse and worse until you just want to hide under the covers until something changes to make you feel better.

You can either wait for something to come along and make the change for you, or you can actively make that change for yourself – and one of the best ways to do that is through gratitude.

In the moments where you're getting down on yourself, take a deep breathe and answer the question, "What am I grateful for right now, in this very moment?"

The answer might be as simple as, "I'm so grateful that I have a comfortable bed in which I can hide until I feel better!"

Gratitude can dig you out of the deepest of holes. It can help you remember that no matter how badly you might be feeling, or how hard on yourself you're being, there are still wonderful, beautiful blessings to enjoy in your life. Life is still good! There is still hope, and it's worth pursuing your best self.

Grace

I've noticed that it's very common for women to get together and talk about what they don't like in their bodies. Whatever it might be, the conversation can easily turn self-deprecating... especially if the topic is the physical body.

Do you ever catch yourself doing that?

As you go about your weight loss journey, notice how you speak about yourself to others. If you're used to making jokes about your thighs, well – cut it out! No more talking about what you don't like about your body, because that kind of language reinforces that sort of thinking, which in turn reinforces a negative self-image. It is so much harder to lose weight when you're down on yourself all the time, and curbing your language is such an easy fix. Much easier – and a great starting point – than changing your internal dialogue.

Love

Ultimately, it always comes back to love. The weight will come off when you lovingly care for yourself and your body, and no amount of tortuous exercise, restricted diet or negative self-talk can take you even close to where you really want to be.

Because, really, what we all want is a fulfilling life of adventure, passion, health, and vibrant love.

It's there for you, Mama – go claim it!

Action Steps

Notice your self-talk, and notice the way you talk about yourself to others. Is it helpful or harmful? It might be time to make a change.

Quick Tip: When you do catch yourself thinking nasty thoughts about yourself, jot them down! Most of the time they're so outrageous that you might just burst out laughing – and that's a great way to release it and move forward.

10 BONUS

Dry Brushing for Immaculate Health

- How to do it: before you step in the shower, take a boars' hair bristle brush and gently brush toward your heart.
- Start with your limbs, moving toward the heart, until you've covered your entire body.
- This practice will help stimulate your lymph nodes to eliminate toxins as well as slough off dead skin cells.

Drink Green Tea

- Consider switching your coffee to green tea to pack in antioxidants and flush toxins through your body more quickly.

Switch to Natural Skincare

- Most skincare products actually aren't that great for our bodies. Instead of spending hundreds of dollars on drugstore or department store lines, consider making your own skin care. Visit www.SaltandRitual.com for great recipes!

ABOUT THE AUTHOR

Virginia Martin is a film fanatic, fitness instructor and writer based in California with her husband, two children and their golden retriever.